Rita Johnson
203 Shady Brook Ct
M.W.C 73110

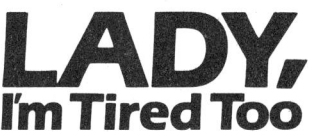

LADY,
I'm Tired Too

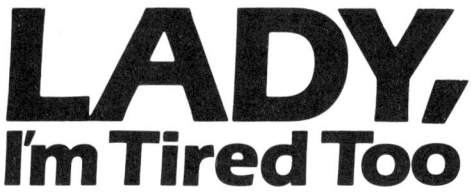

LADY, I'm Tired Too

George E. Vandeman

Pacific Press Publishing Association
Mountain View, California
Oshawa, Ontario

Copyright © 1982 by
Pacific Press Publishing Association
Printed in the United States of America
All Rights Reserved

Cover photo: Glenn Sayers

All biblical quotations, unless otherwise indicated, are from the New International Version

Third Reprinting, 1984

Library of Congress Cataloging in Publication Data

Vandeman, George E.
  Lady, I'm tired too.

  1. Christian life—Adventist authors. I. Title.
BV4501.2.V3295   248.4'8673   81-18890
ISBN 0-8163-0464-5   AACR2

Contents

Lady, I'm Tired Too 9

When Your Number Comes Up 17

The Vegetarian Mystique 26

Just a Puff of Smoke 35

No Bridge to Abraham 45

Hope Gets You Through the Night 55

Have you ever looked up from New York Harbor at the lady with the torch, welcoming the tired and the poor of other lands? Have you ever lifted weary eyes and weary muscles to that silent symbol of liberty and caring, and whispered, "Lady, I'm tired too"?

Lady, I'm Tired Too

When the day has been too long, when the battle has been too much and the bugle too loud and you're tired—too tired—ready to quit—what then?

On one of his programs, Bob Hope reported his activities for the day. He said that his heart beat 103,369 times, and his blood traveled 168 miles. He breathed 23,040 times and inhaled 438 cubic feet of air. He ate three and one fourth pounds of food and drank two pounds of liquid. He perspired one and a half pints. He generated 450 tons of energy. He spoke 4800 words, moved 750 major muscles, and exercised seven million brain cells. And he said, "Boy, am I tired!"

Our civilization is too tense. Too much in a hurry. So concerned with getting there, that it forgets where it is going. It has too many revolving doors, too many committee meetings, and too many telephones.

Someone, in a lighter mood, has pointed out that the bathtub was invented in 1850 and the telephone in 1875. Therefore, if you had been living in 1850, you could have sat in the bathtub for twenty-five years without the phone ringing once!

I didn't check those dates, but the point is made. Life today is too exhausting, too monotonous, too frustrating. Our problems repeat themselves like a jackhammer. The trouble with life, said Dorothy Sayers, is that it's so everlastingly daily!

It gets into our ears after a while, into our nerves, and into our bones. It's no wonder that the most common complaint of our society is "I'm tired!"

Julia Ward Howe is remembered as the author of the words to our beloved "Battle Hymn of the Republic." But once, when it seemed that the weight of the world was upon her, she slumped down in a chair and said that she was tired—"tired way down into the future."

Do you feel like that sometimes?

We need to beware of times like that, because we aren't normal when we're tired. We don't *hear* straight. We take offense at innocent comments never intended to hurt. We don't *see* straight. We see problems that aren't there. And we don't *think* straight. We should never, never make an important decision when we're tired!

There are several brands of tiredness. One of them, familiar to us all, is the *tiredness of physical exhaustion*. And this kind of weariness is easiest of all to fix. A good night's sleep, a little rest, a little relaxation, sitting on a log somewhere watching a waterfall—these will usually do the trick.

When emotional factors are involved in our weariness, it isn't so easy. There is the *tiredness of frustration*. Disappointment. Shattered dreams. Delayed hopes. The eternal waiting for a telephone call that never comes, for a ship to come in, for a knight to come riding.

Rest and relaxation are not much help here. Rest and relaxation too easily turn into giving up and quitting. And that is exactly what the enemy of our souls would be delighted to accomplish. There is an answer to these problems. Disappointments, when we look back from higher ground, are often recognized as among the best of God's favors to us. Shattered dreams are replaced by better ones fulfilled. And delayed hopes are finally a reality. But while we are waiting, it's important not to quit!

You say you're too tired to hang on any longer—you'll have to let go the rope? Well, someone has suggested that that's the trouble with us Christians—the good people get tired being good before the bad people get tired being bad. In other words, what we need is to hang on longer than the devil hangs on—wear him out and get him to quit before he wears us out and gets us to quit.

Single-handed, of course, on our own, we are no match for the once-brilliant angel who turned himself into a devil. But we have divine help—if we ask for it. The apostle Paul says, "No temptation has seized you except what is common to man. And God is faithful; he will not let you be tempted beyond what you can bear. But when you are tempted, he will also provide a way out so that you can stand up under it." 1 Corinthians 10:13.

And the apostle John gives us this encouragement: "The one who is in you is greater than the one who is in the world." 1 John 4:4.

Yes, the Lord Jesus is greater and stronger than all the forces the enemy can array against us. And He's ready to fight our battles for us—our battles against discouragement—if we let Him.

Giving up, letting go the rope—this is the one thing that makes no sense at all. There's a foolish little story that illustrates this:

It's an old story—about the two frogs who fell into a can of cream. They thrashed around and tried their best to hop out. But they couldn't make it. Finally one of the frogs got tired and quit. "What's the use?"

he said. So he flipped his flippers in one last sigh of despair and sank to the bottom.

The other frog was made of sterner stuff. He said, "I may not make it. I, too, may go down. But I'll go down kicking." So he kept kicking, and soon to his surprise, the cream turned to butter. With his feet on a chunk of it, he leaped out.

Well, the apostle Paul makes the point a little more soberly. He says, "And let us not be weary in well doing: for in due season we shall reap, if we faint not." Galatians 6:9, KJV.

If we don't faint. That's the thing!

There's another kind of weariness. It's the *tiredness of depression*. There's a very fine line between tiredness and depression. It's hard to tell which is which—whether you're depressed because you're tired, or tired all the time because you're depressed.

Actually it is perfectly normal to be depressed when you are overtired. But that is temporary. After a good night's sleep you forget you were depressed—or can't remember what you were depressed about.

But sometimes depression takes hold and refuses to let go. Then you're in trouble. A downward spiral begins. You're drenched with pessimism and dark despair. And what to do is the problem.

Emotional depression answers to a variety of names. John Bunyan called it "the slough of despond." The army calls it "battle fatigue." The psychiatrist may label it a "dysthymic disorder." And the layman prefers to speak of it as "nervous exhaustion."

None of these labels were in the vocabulary of David the psalmist, so he simply said, "Out of the depths have I cried unto thee, O Lord," Psalm 130:1, KJV.

And evidently it worked. For David also said, "He brought me up also out of an horrible pit, out of the miry clay, and set my feet upon a rock, and established my goings. And he hath put a new song in my mouth, even praise unto our God." Psalm 40:2, 3, KJV.

The trouble is that too many of us have not cried to the Lord. We have turned everywhere else for help.

Chronic tiredness and depression may have many causes. There may be a physical cause that a careful physician can discover. A problem may need to be talked out with someone qualified to help.

Any number of cures, psychological and physical, have been and are being used for the treatment of depression. And often these are effective. I would not for a moment belittle the work of dedicated psychiatrists. Much good has been done.

However, I am convinced that chronic tiredness and depression are often directly related to an individual's relationship, or lack of relationship, with God. And when that is the case, no therapy that excludes or ignores the spiritual side of man's nature can possibly succeed.

The cure must be appropriate for the disease. Therapy must be directed at the problem. Otherwise it is not therapy. It is wasted time.

If a man has a nail in his foot, it will do no good to X-ray his elbow or scan his brain waves or talk to him about his childhood or give him carrot juice to drink or even put him on crutches. The therapy must be related to the problem. The nail must come out!

Just so, if a man's problem is guilt, he won't be helped by telling him to ignore his conscience and forget the Ten Commandments. That would be like trying to cure a fever by throwing away the thermometer. There is only one cure for guilt, and that is forgiveness. And that is found only at the foot of an old rugged cross!

Could it be that if we would place less dependence

upon cures purchased over the counter and give more attention to strengthening our relationship with our God, we would be able to take the severe stresses that bombard us in this jittery generation?

Some of you may remember a trial that took place back in the fifties. Eleven communist leaders were on trial in New York for conspiracy to overthrow the government by violence. That trial went on for eight months and was presided over by Judge Harold Medina. The behavior of the communists was abominable. They were insolent and arrogant, doing everything in their power to disrupt the proceedings and secure a mistrial. In contrast, Judge Medina exhibited an almost superhuman patience. What was back of this remarkable control? The secret came out when he himself, after the trial was over, told the story of his grueling experience.

Along about the seventh month, he said, he felt he was going to pieces. His nerves were frayed by the constant bickering and by telephone calls threatening his life and the lives of his loved ones. He was on the verge of collapse.

One day he had to leave the courtroom. His head suddenly began to swim. He recessed the court and walked quickly to the little room at the back and lay down. He felt panicky. He was certain he could never go back. He had stood as much as a human being could endure. He knew he would have to quit.

But he said, "Suddenly there in the little room I found myself like a frightened child calling to his father in the dark. I asked God to help me, just to take charge, that His will might be done. I cannot report anything mysterious or supernatural. There was no vision or visitation. All I know is that as I lay on the couch, some new kind of strength flowed into me. I was in that little room for only fifteen minutes, but that brief communion with my God saved not only the trial but my sanity as well. I opened the door and walked again to the bench with a firm realization that I could take whatever was ahead."

What a testimony to the healing power of communion with God! But should it surprise us? Hasn't the Saviour invited the weary, the tired, the burdened, the distressed to come to Him for rest and peace? Listen to His words—and realize that they were intended for you personally, whatever your need:

"Come to me, all you who are weary and burdened, and I will give you rest. Take my yoke upon you and learn from me, for I am gentle and humble in heart, and you will find rest for your souls. For my yoke is easy and my burden is light." Matthew 11:28-30.

What a prescription! For everything that ails us. All our stresses, all our burdens, all our frustrations— yes, all our tears. And then, for good measure, add these words of the Saviour: "Peace I leave with you; my peace I give you. I do not give to you as the world gives. Do not let your hearts be troubled and do not be afraid." John 14:27.

It's a peace that nothing can touch—a peace that no one can take away. With it, we are safe from all the storm and turmoil of the way. Without it, we are easy targets for despair.

Nothing, absolutely nothing, will plunge us into depression more quickly and more surely than separation from our God. We were created for communion with Him. We were never intended to live apart from Him. We will never be truly whole again, truly live again, until the separation is healed!

Sin separates us from God. Only our repentance and His forgiveness can reunite us. Without such a reconciliation, the downward spiral is inevitable. We wander aimlessly along the road to the far country—tired, depressed, tormented with guilt and remorse, knowing that at the end of the road is only famine and despair—while in our Father's house are riches and song!

All the while, walking in the shadows beside us, the Saviour is calling our name. In the night season, when the music stops and the bright lights go out, we hear Him calling us home. He is hurting. We are hurting. We were never meant to be apart. The only way to heal the hurt, to cure the tiredness and loneliness and despair, to quiet the insistent jackhammer of guilt, is to end the separation. You can end it now. And if you do, tomorrow will be better than today!

When Your Number Comes Up

If you stand on seat 22, row 74, section KK, you can look south through the crack and see downtown Oakland. The crack—the width of a clenched fist—cuts through the upper tier of UC Berkeley's Memorial Stadium. And the structure is doomed. It is doomed because this 77,000-seat colossus straddles the Hayward fault—one of the five most dangerous in the country.

Looking south through the crack, you see more than downtown Oakland. You are actually sighting along the approximate course of the Hayward fault. And "along this path of future destruction, north and south, lie 42 schools and hospitals, the Claremont Hotel, BART lines, water tunnels, the El Cerrito fire station—literally thousands of structures, including, ironically, the Alameda County disaster center."— *New West*, August 1981, p. 129.

Has this fault only recently been discovered? No. It was known as early as 1868. Yet few people give it any thought.

What sort of foolishness is it—what sort of fatalism—that leads us to court danger as we do? We march our houses up and down the unstable hillsides. We anchor our bridges in mud. Our proud structures of prestressed concrete are beginning to collapse. So are the instant tilt-ups that pass for buildings in our industrial parks.

Our freeway overpasses easily collapse in a quake. We are told that the Golden Gate Bridge wouldn't go down in a big tremor—but its approaches would.

Now and then a fire, a flood, a mudslide, or an earthquake puts us in our place and shows us how vulnerable we are. But we forget so soon.

Maybe it won't happen, we say. And besides, everyone has to die sometime—*when his number comes up*.

Is it true? Is our future decided in some conference of distant stars—or by the turn of some cosmic roulette wheel? Was the day of our death written into our bodies before we were ever born?

Are our bodies nothing but machines—sophisticated computers into which our behavior has been programmed? Has the human will, our priceless power of choice, been displaced by genes and chromosomes and DNA? And is our health, then, good or bad—is our health only a game in which we are matched against Lady Luck?

A small boy was asked to write an essay about anatomy. This is what he wrote:

"Your head is kind of round and hard and your brains are in it and your hair is on it. Your face is in front of your head where you eat. Your neck is what keeps your head off your shoulders, which are sort of shelves where you hook your overalls suspenders. . . .

"Your arms you got to have to pitch with and so you can reach the biscuits. Your fingers stick out of your hand so you can scratch, throw a curve and add arithmetic. Your legs is what you got to have to get to first base, your feet is what you run on and your toes are what gets stubbed.

"And that is all there is of you except what is inside, and I ain't seen that!"

There has been some disagreement about what is inside!

The Greek philosophers had it all figured out. They said that a man consisted of two parts—a body and a soul. The soul was good and couldn't possibly die. The body was evil and soon to be cast off. Some people still believe this.

But I think you can see that such a belief hardly encourages anyone to take good care of his body. Why should he—if it is evil and soon to be disposed of? It would seem that only spiritual things should demand our attention. And our bodies—aren't they ours to do with as we choose?

Some of you may have wondered why we devote so much time to the subject of health. What possible connection could there be between health and religion? Surely no question of morals is involved in what we eat or drink or how we care for our bodies, you say.

But I'm not so sure. In fact, some of you might be surprised to see how much the Bible has to say about health and the care of our bodies. Would you like just a quick survey? It won't be at all complete, but I think you'll find it both interesting and enlightening.

In the first three chapters of the Bible we find our first parents in a beautiful garden that God has planted especially for them. Fruits and grains and nuts—and later vegetables—are to be their food. Growing in the garden are many trees, already mature, with a large variety of luscious fruits ready to be eaten. And in the center of the garden is the tree of life, the fruit of which is intended to sustain life forever.

One tree, however, is off bounds for the happy couple. And here tragedy enters. For their deliberate disobedience in eating the fruit of the one restricted tree makes it necessary for God to evict them from the garden and bar them from the tree of life.

We move down now to the time of Noah's Flood. After the Deluge, because all vegetation has been destroyed, God permits the eating of the flesh of animals as an emergency measure. But a clear distinction is made between animals fit for food and those not fit for food. You find these restrictions detailed in the eleventh chapter of the book of Leviticus.

As you read the book of Genesis, you notice that the life-span of the human race drops precipitously as soon as the flesh of animals begins to be eaten.

In Abraham's time the city of Sodom is destroyed by fire and brimstone rained down from heaven. And notice what God says through the prophet Ezekiel about the reasons for its destruction. "Now this was the sin of your sister Sodom: She and her daughters were arrogant, overfed and unconcerned. . . . They were haughty and did detestable things before me. Therefore I did away with them as you have seen." Ezekiel 16:49, 50.

Overfed and unconcerned. Do the two go together?

We move on. Esau, one of the sons of Isaac, sells his birthright for a dish of his favorite food.

Then to the time of Moses. God, through Moses, accomplishes what no five-star general today would ever attempt. He moves 600,000 men, besides women and children, on foot through the hot desert—a journey that, because of their lack of faith, takes more than forty years.

How is all this possible? It is possible only because of the laws, the special instructions, that God gives through Moses. Some of these laws concern their diet. Others have to do with the sanitation of campsites, personal cleanliness, the control of communicable diseases, the isolation of lepers, protection of water supplies. And there are many more. It has taken medical science thousands of years to catch up with some of the laws given through Moses.

Still in the Old Testament, we see the young prophet Daniel and three of his friends, Hebrew captives in the city of Babylon, refusing to eat the unhealthful food provided by the king. You find the story in the first chapter of Daniel's book.

Moving over into the New Testament, Zacharias, the father of John the Baptist, receives instruction from an angel about the diet of the son soon to be born.

And now to Jesus Himself. At the very beginning of His public ministry, immediately after His baptism, He goes into the wilderness above the Jordan to fast and pray. And there He meets the most severe temptation possible on the point of appetite—the very point on which our first parents failed.

We see Jesus spending more time in healing than in teaching. There are whole villages where there is not one sick, for He has passed through and healed them all.

When Jesus sends His disciples out into the surrounding country, He commissions them to heal the sick. He himself cannot bear to see anyone hurting, and He wants His disciples to share His compassion.

The apostle James, in the fifth chapter of his letter to fellow Christians, gives us instruction regarding special prayer for the healing of the sick.

But it is the apostle Paul who gives us some of the most helpful counsel on the subject of health. He says, "So whether you eat or drink or whatever you do, do it all for the glory of God." 1 Corinthians 10:31.

The apostle urges us to present our bodies as a living sacrifice to God. He tells us that our bodies are not our own to do with as we choose. Rather, they are intended to be temples in which the Holy Spirit may dwell. Listen: "Do you not know that your body is a temple of the Holy Spirit, who is in you, whom you have received from God? You are not your own; you were bought at a price. Therefore honor God with your body." 1 Corinthians 6:19, 20.

Do you see? If the body is nothing more than an animated machine, soon to be worn out and thrown away, why give it any special care? If it is just a collection of devices for pitching balls and reaching the biscuits, for scratching and adding arithmetic and getting to first base—why not do as we please with it?

But if the body is a temple of the Holy Spirit, if it is not our own, if Jesus has purchased it with His own lifeblood—that changes everything. When this realization comes to a man, he just naturally wants to take care of his body. He wants to keep it in good working condition. He wants to keep it clean. He is careful, now, about what he puts into his body. He will not treat it as a slave. He will not drug it into a dazed limbo of existence.

Health, you see, is not a theory to be discussed. It is not a personal philosophy. No. Just as love is *something we do* in response to another's love—just so, health is *something we do* in response to what our Lord has done for us.

Let's say it another way. Health is not an accident. Health, good or bad, is not determined by some number that suddenly pops up with our name on it. It is not decided by where some cosmic roulette wheel stops. Our health, most of the time—with certain exceptions of course—is determined by what we *have done or not done* about the laws of health—by our own action or inaction.

Every act, or failure to act, carries with it certain consequences. When we choose an act, we are agreeing to attend the banquet of consequences that is sure to follow. We may not like the menu. But we'll be there!

It is a law of health, a law of nature, a law of the universe, that we reap what we sow. The apostle Paul said it this way: "Do not be deceived: God cannot be mocked. A man reaps what he sows." Galatians 6:7.

The hospitals are filled with people who are reaping what they have sown.

The man who smokes for thirty years and then gets lung cancer may be hard put to find anything positive in his experience. He may have stopped his smoking a full year ago, and he wonders why God doesn't step in and spare him from the consequences of those thirty years.

Yet that man, along with all others who are reaping an unpleasant harvest—that man, if he will, may find some comfort in the thought that he is contributing to the stability of the universe.

What do I mean? Simply this. As I said a moment ago, it is a law of the universe, a law of God's government, that a man reaps what he sows. But a government whose laws are only randomly enforced commands no respect. If God were to let too many of us off the hook, if He were to intervene too often to override the law of cause and effect and spare us from the consequences of our wrong choices—which is exactly what He would *like* to do for His children in *every* instance—we wouldn't have much respect for His laws, would we? And where respect for law breaks down, anarchy and chaos are sure to follow.

Some of you, reading this just now, may be scheduled, tomorrow morning, to take that fast and frightening ride by gurney, down the hall and through the double doors to the place where doctors wait in their surgery greens. Or you may now be recovering, slowly and painfully, from such an experience.

Take some comfort, if you will, in the fact that by demonstrating, however reluctantly, the certainty and consistency of God's laws, you are contributing to the stability of His universe.

Take comfort too—greater comfort—in knowing that God cares. He loves you. He has not forgotten you. Somewhere in the shadows, silent and unseen, He is sharing this difficult experience with you.

But right here I'd like to tell you a story. I've told it before. But some stories deserve more than one telling.

Nine-year-old Tommy, wet and bedraggled in his angel costume and yellow wig, sat in a tree not far from the bridge that might collapse at any moment. He had been at the school, practicing for the Easter pageant. He hadn't wanted to go. After all, what nine-year-old boy wants to be cast as an angel with wings and yellow curls? But his mother had insisted.

On the way home a violent storm had come up. Tommy knew that the bridge could not be trusted in a storm. It was one that a group of neighbors had built to save going ten miles around the lake. His father had told him, in a situation like this, just to climb a tree and wait for him to come after him. So Tommy waited.

Through the dense fog he saw lights approaching. As the car came into view, he saw that it was old Sandy McPherson. None of the neighbors had ever seen Sandy sober. If he had been drinking now—and he almost certainly had—he might not use good judgment. He might drive onto the precarious bridge.

So Tommy called out as loudly as he could, "Sandy, don't take the bridge! Go around the lake!"

Tommy started to climb down, for surely Sandy would take him home. But Sandy took off as if he had seen a ghost!

A few minutes later Tommy's father, on his way to pick up his boy, met Sandy on the road. Sandy got out of his car—pale, his lips quivering, his hands shaking. For the first time in anyone's memory, he was cold sober. "You won't believe me," he gasped, "but I just saw a vision! God hasn't forgotten me! The good God—He hasn't forgotten!"

Tommy's father tried to calm him. "Take a deep breath and tell me slowly. You must get hold of yourself."

"Well, I'd had a few drops of whiskey, to keep the chill off, you understand. It was getting dark and the visibility was zero. I was about to turn onto the bridge when I heard a voice say, 'Sandy, don't take the bridge! Go around the lake!' "

Sandy continued, still out of breath. "I looked up, and there, floating between the trees, was an angel! Dressed in white he was, with wings on his shoulders, and yellow curls on his head!"

"What did you do?"

"I threw my bottle out with all my force. If the good God thinks enough of old Sandy McPherson to send an angel to warn him, I won't be a party to destroying myself!"

And Sandy McPherson was never known to take another drink. Throwing his bottle away was something he wanted to *do* for his Lord because of what his Lord had done for him.

All a mistake, you say? Not an angel around? Maybe so. But I'm not so sure God didn't arrange it all, just that way!

Is there something you want to do for *your* Lord—maybe throwing something away? Something that's been destroying you?

The Vegetarian Mystique

Fads—and bandwagons—come and go. A big flash—and then they are gone. Is the present popularity of the vegetarian diet destined soon to fade away—like a politician who doesn't quite make it at the ballot box?

Americans, in a growing distrust of the establishment, sent a peanut farmer to the White House. And Washington menus blossomed with peanut dishes: peanut salads, peanut soup, peanut desserts. Peanut snacks. Peanut-butter sandwiches. Even peanut-butter milkshakes—which I'm told are delicious.

Then, with a new president, came the jelly-bean revival. Jelly-beans—and decorative jelly-bean containers—everywhere.

Now peanuts—in moderation—are good food. But the high sugar content of jelly-beans would hardly recommend them for a place in nutrition's hall of fame.

Even so, I would rather trust high-level decisions made over a jar of jelly-beans than those made in a smoke-filled room. Minds would be *a little* clearer.

But vegetarianism isn't a fad. It isn't going to go away. It has been around for a long time and has survived many a slump—and experienced many a revival—through the ages.

Actually, the earliest record of a vegetarian diet is

found in the Bible, in the very first chapter. God said to the man He had just created, "I give you every seed-bearing plant on the face of the whole earth and every tree that has fruit with seed in it. They will be yours for food." Genesis 1:29.

That's interesting. Fruits, grains, and nuts—later vegetables. But no flesh food. This was the diet chosen by the Creator for the human race.

I well remember the first car I ever bought—my first *new* car, that is. (My first *car* cost me only thirty-five dollars.) I was still a late teenager, and I drove this shiny automobile out of the showroom and round the block—ever so carefully. Then I stopped and took out the owner's manual, to see what the manufacturer recommended. What kind of fuel, what kind of oil, how much air in the tires. I tell you, a car never had better care than that one!

But let me ask you, If a manufacturer knows best what to put in a *car*, don't you suppose the Creator knew best what to put into the *people* He had made?

So there was a time, you see, when everybody on this planet was a vegetarian. And evidently they thrived on it, for those antediluvians had a life-span of hundreds of years. Adam himself lived for 930 years, and Methuselah lived 969 years.

It wasn't until after the Flood of Noah's day, when every living thing had been destroyed and there was literally nothing on earth to eat—it wasn't until then that God gave permission for the flesh of animals to be eaten. Even then it was not an unrestricted permission. Only certain animals, which God designated as clean, were to be eaten. And the blood was first to be drained from the carcass. It was never to be consumed.

Did you ever eat a steak without the blood? Well, you'd soon find something else to eat, for it's the blood that gives it its characteristic flavor.

Now the interesting thing is this. Immediately after the Flood, when the human race turned to a diet of flesh food, life-span took a nose dive. Is there some connection? Personally, I believe that God permitted the eating of the flesh of animals not only as an emergency measure, but also *in order* to shorten men's life-spans. Never again, as before the Flood, would brilliant minds be able to pursue their evil designs for centuries. Think, if you will, what would happen if the inventive minds of a Thomas Edison and an Alexander Graham Bell, urged on by a Hitler, were to devote themselves to the building of nuclear weapons—and had centuries to perfect their lethal projects! No reflection on either Edison or Bell, of course—even if I did put them in bad company!

Well, moving on down—the Egyptians raised cereal grains from the earliest times and were nicknamed "eaters of the bread." Studies of the mummies indicate that their diet consisted primarily of plant foods.

This was not always the case in Egypt, however. For the book of Numbers tells us that the Hebrews who escaped from Egypt under the leadership of Moses longed for the fleshpots of Egypt. In fact, they complained so bitterly that God caused a strong wind to drive quail in from the sea, until they were three feet deep around the camp. But it was not a happy feast, for many of the people died.

"It is interesting," says *Life and Health* magazine, "that the dietary patterns of nations pass through various well-defined stages. When a nation is struggling to grow and its people are poor, the diet is usually frugal, consisting chiefly of plant foods. As prosperity increases, animal foods and wine become more plentiful. Later, self-indulgence and decay set in. Philosophers of every age who observed these trends concluded that they led to the downfall of nations." So it is no surprise that those arose who advocated a return to a more simple diet.

Although they were not strict vegetarians themselves, the Greek philosophers Pythagoras, Socrates, and Plato popularized the idea and supported such a program.

And of course Buddhism, Brahmanism, and Hinduism all extol a vegetarian diet, though those who do not adhere to it are not penalized.

Did you know that John Wesley, the famed pioneer of the Methodist Church, was a vegetarian? And Charles Spurgeon of London, the Billy Graham of the last century? Benjamin Franklin was a great promoter of the vegetarian diet. And George Bernard Shaw.

Even Shakespeare must have understood some of these things. For he put these words into the mouth of Falstaff the fool: "I am a great lover of meat; sometimes methinks 'tis that which makes me wits so dull."

A story that I have told before is so appropriate that it must be told again. It's an old story about a science professor in a boys' school. He had an uncanny knowledge of animal life. You could show him the bone of an animal, and he would identify it. Animal life was his world.

One day the boys decided to play a little trick on the professor. They took the skeleton of a bear and stuffed it. Then they sewed over it the skin of a lion. On its head they fastened the horns of a Texas steer, and on its feet they glued the hoofs of a wild buffalo.

They spent a good many nights on the trick, and they did a pretty good job. Then one afternoon when the professor was taking a nap, they tiptoed into his study and set up the monstrosity. And finally, from outside the door, they let out an unearthly growl such as had never been heard before.

The professor woke up, the story says, tumbled off his cot, and stood bolt upright. His reaction was enough to justify all the time they had spent on the trick. But then through their peepholes they saw a surprising thing. The professor rubbed his eyes, looked at the teeth, the horns, and finally at the split hoofs. Then he said, loud enough for the peepholers to hear, "Thank goodness! It's herbivorous, not carnivorous!" And he went back to finish his nap.

The professor knew that any animal with horns and split hoofs is a vegetarian and would prefer hay or grass to a sleeping professor!

How do *you* react to a *person* who is a vegetarian? If you are like most people, you probably consider him harmless, even if you do think he is strangely put together—and go back to your nap.

People become vegetarians for a variety of reasons. Some, of course, make the change because of the high cost of meat. Some for health reasons. Some because they feel that the slaughter of animals for food is morally wrong. And some see the vegetarian way of life as part of an attempt to escape from our mechanized society.

Susan St. James has an interesting angle. She strongly believes that you can tell a vegetarian by his disposition. She says, "There's a calm that comes over you and a tremendous peace of mind when you're around vegetarians."

Do you suppose vegetarians really are more comfortable to be around? I would hope so, of course—since I happen to be one!

To be more exact, I am a lacto-ovo-vegetarian. That simply means that my diet is one that includes a moderate amount of dairy products. And the vegetarian diet, in my experience—in my own home and around the world—has been associated with gracious and delightful dining.

But you say, "Surely you can't expect a working man to turn out a hard day's work on nothing but bread, beans, and bananas."

Well, why not? In the animal kingdom the real beasts of burden eat only plants. The big killer cat is good for short bursts of energy. But that's all.

It was Teddy Roosevelt who said that if you hitch a lion to a plow, he would soon fall from exhaustion. But the horse can plow all day long!

Henry Thoreau once visited a farmer plowing his field with a team of oxen. As the two men walked behind the plow, they talked about the kind of diet best suited to build strong bodies. The farmer said, "You cannot live on vegetable foods solely, for they furnish nothing to build bones with."

And Henry Thoreau mused, "All the while he talks he is walking behind his oxen which with vegetable-made bones jerk him and his plow along."

You see, endurance is the test. And it's carbohydrate primarily, not protein, that gives you staying power. Nutritionists know now that we don't need anywhere near as much protein as was once thought.

A Swedish scientist tested nine trained athletes on a stationary bicycle. They were to pump the pedals until their legs would no longer respond. But first, before being tested, these athletes were put on a high fat and protein diet—that is, meat, eggs, fish, cheese, etc.—for three days. Then they pedaled the stationary bike. But they ran out of steam in an average of fifty-seven minutes.

Then those very same athletes were put on a mixed diet such as most people eat—for three days. They were able to pedal twice as long—an average of 114 minutes.

But now listen. These same men were then put on a low protein, high carbohydrate diet—high in vegetables and grains—for three days. This time they were able to hold out for an average of 167 minutes—almost three times as long as on the largely meat diet!

Is it any wonder that so many athletes are vegetarians? They know where to turn for real go power, real staying power.

Many people have the idea that our bodies are intended for a meat diet, that anything else is somehow strange and unnatural. But nothing could be farther from the truth. The Creator included no flesh food at all in the diet He personally selected and provided for the human race. Remember?

A careful study of man's digestive apparatus clearly shows that he is not well equipped to handle a flesh diet. He is obviously designed to subsist on vegetarian foods. Yet he has perverted his dietary habits to accept the food of the carnivore.

Mahatma Gandhi, a committed vegetarian, once said, "I hold flesh food to be unsuited to our species." And he added, "We err in copying the lower animal world—if we are superior to it."

One of the best reasons for being a vegetarian today is the tremendous increase of disease—especially cancer—in animals, in fish, and in fowl. And what assurance do we have that the cancer virus in animals cannot be transferred to humans?

You say, "The meat is all inspected, so it's safe."

Yes, it's inspected. But I'm not so sure it's safe.

Tell me. Do you know how many human bodies a pathologist inspects in a day? Probably not more than three or four. And he never works without a microscope.

But you see, there aren't enough veterinarians to do the inspecting of meat, so lay people with very little training are utilized. And often these lay inspectors are asked to examine a hundred or more cattle in a day. And without a microscope!

Do you see? Aside from the debate about how careful the inspectors are or aren't, their assignment is an impossible one!

What happens if a cancer *is* discovered—one too obvious to miss? Sometimes, of course, the entire animal is discarded. But there is documented evidence that all too often the cancer is simply cut away and the rest of the animal sold for food. Do you really want to eat a piece of meat that has shared circulating blood with a cancer?

And here is something else. Did you ever hear of benzopyrene? Did you know that in a little over two pounds of charcoal-broiled steak there's as much benzopyrene—a cancer-stimulating agent—as in the smoke from six hundred cigarettes? Did you get that? That steak on the barbecue—a benzopyrene risk equal to thirty packs of cigarettes!

It's true that the benzopyrene from cigarette smoke is inhaled, while in the steak it is eaten. Wouldn't that make a difference? Probably so. You might get cancer of the stomach instead of cancer of the lung!

We are all economy-minded these days—by necessity. We have to use our resources wisely. So one more thing. Suppose that you have a piece of land. How can you best use it? You can grow food crops for human consumption. Or you can grow food for animals, and feed the animals to the people. Do you realize that you can feed fourteen times as many people with that piece of land if you simply grow food crops for humans?

Or put it this way. If you put one hundred calories into the cow, you get four calories out. In other words, you get back in beef just one twenty-fifth of the calories you fed the cow. Not very good planning, is it?

Wouldn't it be smarter to eat the plants yourself?

You say, "I'm convinced. But I wouldn't have the slightest idea how to prepare a vegetarian meal. I need help!"

There are, of course, a great many prepared foods available today, and some of them are very acceptable. Our space-age technology, especially the spun-fiber technique, has made it possible to duplicate both the texture and flavor of meat. These prepared entrées will be a help to you in making a smooth transition to a more healthful diet.

I think just one meal at our house would convince you that it isn't any sacrifice at all to be a vegetarian. My wife Nellie is a master at preparing light and delicious vegetarian entrées that you would never forget. Put one of them with a baked potato, a green salad, a light dessert, some homemade whole-wheat bread. And you'll be wanting more!

I say again, it isn't any sacrifice at all to be a vegetarian. It's just another step toward the radiant health you've always wanted—the health God wants you to have. It's just another step toward an unblemished skin, a new spring in your step, a new light in the eye. It's a step toward untroubled sleep and a new vigor in the morning.

It's just another step toward an unclouded mind and clear decisions. It's just another step toward being ready for a world where there is no death. No death for anyone. For anything. Ever!

Just a Puff of Smoke

A single match—in the hand of a San Francisco painter. The tiny flame flickered for a moment—as if reluctant to fulfill its deadly mission.

But the hand that held it was determined. The match had been struck in anger—and revenge. The painter had hidden his equipment here while taking a break at a neighborhood saloon. And now his tools were gone. Maybe this would show them—whoever "them" might be!

There was a puff of smoke. And then—the flames became a raging inferno as the workman ran in terror from what his hands had done. It wasn't just a fire. It was a conflagration surpassed in San Francisco only by the fires that accompanied the 1906 earthquake. Twenty-seven buildings were destroyed or badly damaged before it was brought under control.

And it all started with a revengeful thought, a single match, and a reluctant puff of smoke!

Jerry Scribner woke up from a bad dream. It was so lacking in drama that it hardly seems worth telling. He dreamed that he walked into his office, and his staff showed him a map marking three thousand locations where fly larvae had been found.

That's humdrum, you say. But wait. The larvae

were those of the Mediterranean fruit fly. And Jerry Scribner was director of the Medfly project. To him it was a very bad dream!

And it wasn't many weeks till Jerry Scribner began to wonder if the dream may have been prophetic. For California was struggling with its greatest crisis in years. Its multi-billion-dollar agricultural industry was threatened by the tiny Medfly. And here was not a problem for flyswatters. It would take a swat team from the sky—helicopters or bombers armed with malathion, which people, along with the bugs, must breathe.

And so, while men argued and procrastinated and blamed, trying to please the farmers and the environmentalists at one and the same time, the area of infestation grew with breathtaking speed. The Medfly was already out of control, some said. And probably no man in California carried so heavy a weight on his shoulders, while everybody watched, as Jerry Scribner, assigned to get rid of the fly. It's no wonder it filled his mind and spilled over into his dreams!

Actually, California's battle with the Medfly is only the latest skirmish in an agelong conflict with our tiny competitors, the insects.

"We are not the dominant life form on earth," said Roger Caras, ABC's wildlife correspondent. "Insects not only outnumber us to an astronomical degree, they outlive us."

"There is nothing strong enough that we know of to control them for any length of time that we can tolerate ourselves. Because there is no way of building a wall between the insects and us. They use the same air, the same moisture that we do, they live in the same habitats we do."

"One problem is their short life. They reproduce [more rapidly than we can cope with them]. We invent a poison, only to find that in a matter of months, or at the most a few years . . . [they are devouring the poison] as if it were a treat."

"We don't even have the option of killing all the insects. Our agriculture would suffer irreparable harm, for . . . many of the plants we eat require insects to pollinate them. If the insects are ever destroyed, one way or another, they will take us with them. . . . Insects have more power over us than we have over them. Insects are a science fiction movie come true!"

Yes, California's most stubborn crisis in years began with a single Medfly—and a single apricot. Or was it a plum?

I wonder if we realize how often our future depends upon little things—little acts, little decisions. Going through a door. Choosing one path over another.

It was Solomon the wise man who said, "There is a way that seems right to a man, but in the end it leads to death." Proverbs 14:12.

We may not intend to spend much time on the path that seems so enchanting. We just want to try it out, investigate it, see what it is like. We forget that it only takes a moment to step into the popular traffic. But it's a long way back—if ever we have the opportunity to come back!

Kansas City was proud of its Hyatt Regency. It was two structures really—joined by its lobby. And overlooking the lobby—an architectural feature that made it unique—were three sky bridges. Even during the day it was something to see and remember. Staircases appearing out of nowhere. Lights shining down from the ceiling. Trees growing from the floor. The front and back walls entirely of glass.

The 40-story, 750-room hotel had been open only a year. The Friday-evening tea dances, introduced six weeks earlier, had proved to be immensely popular. On this night there were at least 2000 people present, most of them dancing on the lobby floor. Probably 50 were dancing or watching from the fourth-floor skybridge, and about 200 from the suspended walkway at second-floor level.

Suddenly, without time to run or scream, it happened. The fourth-floor skybridge buckled and fell onto the second-floor walkway, and both collapsed onto the dancing crowd below. One moment it was a party atmosphere. The next moment death was on the loose. When the count was in it would be 114 dead, 186 hurt, with ten lifted out uninjured.

The difference between life and death that fateful night was measuared in seconds—and in inches.

Ann Dunford had one foot on the second-level skywalk. She doesn't know if she felt it give, or heard it. But she stepped back, fell—but got up and walked away.

Sandy Goodrick and three friends entered the hotel about five minutes before the collapse. Two of her friends were trapped in the rubble.

Matthew Stevenson, an associate editor of *Harper's* magazine, was also there—not by design, but by accident. Arriving just after it happened, he was told the building was off limits to everybody, especially the press. But by way of a fire escape and a stairwell, he managed to reach the ledge of the upper skybridge, the one that had collapsed. He says:

"My knees literally shook and buckled as I crept clinging to the wall, down the short hallway that led to the open space.

"Where once there had been a promenade 100 feet in the air across a gracious lobby there was now only a void. Between myself and the other side were only the cries of the injured and the dying from the abyss below."

For more than ten hours he watched from his little perch as firemen and policemen—with the skill and the care of archaeologists—"uncovered what seemed like a generation trapped between two collapsed walkways."

He says, "The bodies I saw rescue workers drag out one by one in horrifying slow motion seemed stopped in time, as if they had been frozen by lightning.

"A woman in white high heels held her hand, now fixed by rigor mortis, to her cheek, as if still flirting with a dance partner. An elderly black man . . . had the look of someone on his way to dinner. . . . There were whole clusters of persons obviously chatting amiably during the dance when the sword fell, and they all died in place."

He concludes, "If a few survived, many were not so lucky. They were in the wrong place. Period. There was no wrong time because it was over in an instant."—*San Francisco Sunday Examiner and Chronicle*, July 19, 1981.

Makes you think of Pompeii, doesn't it?

How could such an accident happen—in so new and modern a structure? What caused it? We may never know. But experts, some of them engineers, suspect that foot-tapping revelers, their bodies swaying with the music, may have touched off a deadly vibration that caused the walkways to collapse in an avalanche of concrete and steel.

Think of it! Such a little thing as tapping feet—playing into the hands of death!

Sir Walter Raleigh. Remember that name? He was a favorite of Queen Elizabeth I. And whether or not he placed his cloak in the mud for her, he must have had personal charm.

But did you know that this same dashing and talented Sir Walter Raleigh had much to do with establishing tobacco and the tobacco habit on both sides of the Atlantic?

It is said that his servant, the first time he saw him smoking, drenched his master with water to save him from burning.

Nevertheless, it was this dashing and talented Walter Raleigh, hooked by the habit, who took tobacco from Virginia to England, and no product ever received a more immediate and overwhelming acceptance. James I, who had succeeded Elizabeth I, wrote a special tract against the use of tobacco, but nothing could stop the spread of the habit.

It is no surprise that the king and Sir Walter were not friends. After a long series of conflicts with the crown, Raleigh was given the death sentence. But as a last gesture of defiance to the king, it is said that he puffed a pipe of tobacco before ascending the scaffold to die.

Yes, how often a puff of smoke has been the expression of inner feelings, of inner frustration. Teenage feelings of defiance—of rebellion—reacting to peer pressure—wanting to appear grown-up—not wanting to be chicken.

And how often a puff of smoke, under the cover of sophistication, has expressed the desperation of millions of adults who would gladly quit—if only they could!

Big disasters don't usually start big. They start small. A little rain. Then more and more. The quiet little creeks become torrents—the rivers are swollen. And finally the disaster headlines. And it all began with a single drop of rain!

At least 75,000 personal disasters—fatal tragedies—touch and sadden the families of our nation every year. Tragedies that began with just a puff of smoke!

These personal tragedies, lives lost in their prime, didn't happen immediately, in a few terrifying seconds, as at the Hyatt Regency. That first cigarette caused no conflagration to rival the fires of San Francisco's 1906.

Death was working slowly, subtly, constantly assuring its victims that everything was all right, that tragedy would never touch them as it had thousands of others. There was plenty of time. They could smoke another five years and still have time to quit. Yet death had been in control from the moment of that first puff of smoke. And men and women, boys and girls, had been its slaves.

Lincoln freed the slaves. Yes. But he didn't free them all. For the weed that Sir Walter promoted has made more slaves than ever picked cotton in the South. It has taken a toll greater than all our wars.

The cruel and ruthless damage has not been done in the dark, foul-smelling holds of slave ships. It has not been done at the hands of uncaring plantation owners. No. The hand of death takes its toll in the halls where laws are made, in committee rooms where strategies are perfected, in the homes of the rich and the famous—and wherever there is a puff of smoke.

Millions, since the days of Sir Walter, have thought they were strong, have thought they were in control. They could stop anytime. But they *didn't*—because they *couldn't*. They were slaves to a puff of smoke!

It does little good to recite the horrors of lung cancer to the smoker in your life. He knows them all by heart. And besides, how can the reality—the dimension of the danger—get through to the mind that is dulled by the weed to which he is addicted?

Every puff of smoke is a decision. But it is a decision made by a mind that is progressively less able to make wise decisions. Smoke is hazing up the mind that must call for help!

Such is the subtle trickiness of a puff of smoke! Is it

any wonder that Satan, the fallen angel, the enemy of us all, as he planned his strategy to destroy us—is it any wonder that he settled on that which would dull the mind, and with it the conscience?

If only commercials would tell the truth! You can keep on smoking, they imply. Just use the toothpaste that gets your teeth whiter and whiter—while your lungs are getting blacker and blacker.

The commercials always picture that puff of smoke in the setting of spring and sophistication. Spring and springtime air, untainted by the product they sell.

They don't tell you the heartbreak of losing one you love to the ugly weed. They don't show you the pitiful scars. They don't show you the victims of emphysema gasping for breath—victims of a puff of smoke.

Our government acted so promptly with cranberries—and soup. It wouldn't want to see one person die needlessly. But with one hand it blesses no-smoking campaigns, while with the other it subsidizes the farmers growing tobacco. How hypocritical can we be?

It may not be smoking that is your problem. It may be drugs or drink or whatever. It may be money that is your god. Or it may be food. Judas sold his Lord for thirty pieces of silver. But some of us have sold Him for a scoop of ice cream. Miserable bargain!

"Do not be deceived: God cannot be mocked. A man reaps what he sows." Galatians 6:7.

It works with mathematical precision. It works every time. Is it any wonder that Jesus struggled forty days in the wilderness to gain, for you and me, the victory over appetite? And because He did, there is hope!

Just a puff of smoke. Just like any other puff of smoke. It lingers a moment and is gone. But if that puff of smoke is a symbol of deadly procrastination, from a heart that really wants to quit, then that puff of smoke is different. It is a call for help!

And leaping from the Book is just the help you need. Listen to this: "Sin shall not have dominion over you." Romans 6:14, KJV.

There it is! You don't have to sin! You don't have to smoke! You don't have to treat your body so!

The little weed may be tightening its grip. It may have more power over you than you have over it. But that control can be broken. You don't have to wait for that elusive, perfect day when you can walk up to a pack of cigarettes like a hero—all on your own—and throw them away forever. That day never comes!

But the Lord Jesus came to set the captives free. And listen: "If the Son sets you free, you will be free indeed." John 8:36.

When the Lord Jesus slices the sky with a brilliance and a thunder such as we have never dreamed, when all nature is in upheaval and it seems the earth is breaking up, when every man and woman knows that time is gone forever, many will be found still tightly clutching a puff of smoke. And I say again, What a miserable bargain!

And you say, "Evidently I can't go into my Lord's presence like this. I have to stop smoking first."

No, friend, you don't. The truth is that you probably *can't* stop smoking first. You need a Saviour first. Then He can lift you out of the polluted air. He can break the chains of those intangible, worthless, hypnotic puffs of smoke. He'll gladly do it now—if you'll let Him. You can walk out into the sunshine free—in His power, not your own!

You may be weak. You may think you have no willpower left. But you can still choose. You can still call for help.

Listen, friend, whoever you are and wherever you

are, Jesus knows your weakness. He knows every circumstance of your life. But He loves you all the more because of your weakness.

Just as a mother loves the sick child more, just as the shepherd leaves his ninety-nine in the fold and goes to search for the one that is lost—just so Jesus is nearest to those who need Him most. He saves His finest miracle for His weakest child!

And that miracle—the miracle of a new life—can be yours just now—before you turn the page!

No Bridge to Abraham

Bridges! They fascinate us. The George Washington Bridge, thrown like a drawbridge across the Hudson from upper Manhattan to the New Jersey cliffs. Slung with 105,000 miles of cable!

Scenic bridges like the one at Bixby Creek, spanning Big Sur's wild and rocky landscape as it rises almost vertically out of the Pacific Ocean!

The San Francisco-Oakland Bay Bridge, stretching, with its approaches, for eight miles!

And the Golden Gate Bridge—constructed where it was said a bridge could not be built. But it was. And its single, 4200-foot span is one of the most spectacular engineering feats of all time!

Bridge-builders are only challenged by the yawning chasms that are called *impassable*. They dream their impossible dreams and make them come true. Only the ocean holds them back. And they are working on bridging it!

But one man, according to a story that Jesus told, found himself on the wrong side of a gulf that no engineer could bridge—even by dreaming very, very hard!

Why did Jesus so often speak in parables? Why didn't He come right out and say what He wanted to say?

And what is a parable? I like the way David Redding has explained it. "A fable," he says, "is a fantastic tale with trees and foxes speaking. A proverb is a statement with no tale at all. An allegory is a story with each part robotlike, standing for something. But a parable is a story true to this house of earth, but with a window open to the sky."

Parables are not meant for theologians. They are for the people. They are not meant to be dissected and analyzed, trying to find some meaning in every word. They are not necessarily true to fact in every detail. If you wish to discover the true teaching of the Bible, do not try to find it in the details of a parable.

A parable, you see, is an imaginary story meant to put across a point. Our aim should be to find its point, its big idea, and then, as someone has said, "be not overbusy about the rest."

It was stubborn hearts that Jesus was especially trying to reach with the stories He told. Truth hidden in a parable could slip in unnoticed, go straight to its target, and then burst into bloom when it was too late to keep it out.

The enemies of Jesus resisted truth. But they would listen to a story. Stories were safe. They were about somebody else. And again and again they were led to condemn themselves before they realized that they themselves were the villains.

Jesus was not trying to lock truth away from anyone. Rather, He was trying to break the lock on hardened hearts He could reach in no other way. And many a man, caught up in the story, was stirred to belief before he realized he had been struck.

Jesus told a story one day about a rich man and a beggar. And He put into it something that most men never see until the day they know they are going to die.

The rich man, He said, lived in luxury. And the

beggar at his gate lived on crumbs from the rich man's table.

The rich man was not one who openly declared his disregard for God and man. He claimed to be a true son of Abraham. The sight of the beggar at his gate was repulsive. But he showed no violence toward him. He didn't curse him. He didn't ask his servants to take him away. He gained a certain satisfaction from the fact that the crumbs from his table—delivered each day by his order, no doubt—were keeping the poor beggar alive.

Beyond that the rich man felt no further responsibility. He was selfishly indifferent to the needs of the beggar at his gate. He was aloof, neutral, untouched—and felt no guilt. The beggar ought to be glad for the crumbs. And undoubtedly he was.

But one day, according to the story, the beggar died. And so did the rich man. Lazarus, the beggar, was carried by the angels into Abraham's bosom. And the rich man arrived in hell.

Now, the details of this story were never intended to give an accurate picture of what happens at death. Certainly Abraham's bosom could never hold all the good people who ever lived. Neither is this the place to look for a literal description of hell.

Pushing aside, then, any concern about the details, the point of the story is as clear as the noonday sun. In the future life some roles will be reversed. There will be some big surprises when we see who goes where. The poor beggar finds himself in the company of Abraham. And the rich man—who is proud to be a descendant of Abraham and depends upon that relationship—is completely shut away from Abraham.

Now what happens? The story says that the rich man, tormented in the flames of hell, looks up and sees Abraham far away, with the beggar at his side. And he calls out to him, "Father Abraham, have pity on me and send Lazarus to dip the tip of his finger in water and cool my tongue, because I am in agony in this fire."

But Abaraham replies, "Son, remember that in your lifetime you received your good things, while Lazarus received bad things, but now he is comforted here and you are in agony. And besides all this, between us and you a great chasm has been fixed, so that those who want to go from here to you cannot, nor can anyone cross over from there to us." Luke 16:24-26.

Again, the details here were never intended to be taken literally. Certainly heaven and hell would not be such close proximity that the saved and the lost can call back and forth and communicate. Heaven would hardly be a place to be desired if the torment of those in hell, perhaps including some loved ones, could be both seen and heard.

But the points of the story, the messages Jesus put into the story, fairly shout. Some roles, in the future life, will be reversed. There will be some surprises. But those roles, those destinations, will have been decided here, in this life. And there will be no appeal. There will be no second chance. Because a great chasm has been fixed, an impassable gulf, between the saved and the lost. And no engineer in heaven or hell can build a bridge across it. There will be no bridge to Abraham for those who have not lived the life and shown the faith of Abraham!

Yes, a great chasm is fixed between the saved and the lost. And it is fixed, irreversibly fixed, in this life, not in the next. And once it is fixed, no man can cross it. There is no bridge to Abraham!

The resurrection is held out, all through the Bible, as the hope of the Christian. And what a day it will be! The crippled will walk, and the dumb will shout for joy. There will be no blind eyes and no ears that cannot hear. Confused minds will never be confused again. And the weary will thrill with the vigor of eternal youth!

The resurrection day will be a day of miracles for every child of God. Pain and tears and death will be no more. For each one will receive from his Lord a new body—a body not subject to death. What a day!

But there is one miracle that will not be worked on that day. And that is the miracle of character transformation. The resurrection will not change any man's character. When the voice of the Saviour calls the dead to life, they will come from the grave with the same appetites and passions, the same likes and dislikes, as in this life.

The moment of resurrection will change men physically, but not morally. The criminal who in the last moment of life was bent on crime, will still be bent on crime when he awakes. Each mind will pick up where it left off. The man who hated God will still hate Him. The man who took no pleasure in the company of God's people in this life will shun their company in the next. His own desires and choices will either fit him for heaven or eternally shut him out. God will not force him to change his mind!

Those of God's children who are still living when Jesus appears in the skies will enter the new life without passing through death. The apostle Paul says, "Listen, I tell you a mystery: We will not all sleep, but we will all be changed—in a flash, in the twinkling of an eye, at the last trumpet. For the trumpet will sound, the dead will be raised imperishable, and we will be changed. For the perishable must clothe itself with the imperishable, and the mortal with immortality." 1 Corinthians 15:51-53.

What a moment that will be! But that moment will

make no character change. The transformation of character that makes a man a safe candidate for immortality, for life that never ends, will have been made in this life. There is nothing about translation that will change the bent of his mind. The man who goes glibly along, tolerating his sins, satisfied that the moment of translation will take away his bent to sinning and fit him for heaven—that man will be sadly disappointed.

Now I know that not one of us can ever overcome sin in our own strength. It will take a miracle. But the Lord Jesus wants to work that miracle for us now. If we are not willing to accept that miracle now, He will not impose it upon us then!

Thousands are waiting for some magic bridge by which they can change sides at the last moment. But it will never happen. They are dreaming an impossible dream!

There will be no miracle at the last moment to change men's characters. And neither will there be a miracle at the last to change men's *appetites*. Have you ever thought about that?

Jesus, here on earth, loved people. He loved to be with them. He was often present at the banquets they prepared. And some of the stories He told have to do with banquets, feasts, weddings.

He told about the man who prepared a banquet and invited his guests, but they would not come. He wanted us to know that all are welcome in His kingdom. All are invited. Those who are left out are left out by their own choice.

He told about the guest who went to a wedding without the wedding garment that was provided. That garment is the righteousness of Christ. But the guest refused it. He chose to depend on his own good works. Or, like the rich man in the story we've been discussing, he chose to depend upon his blood relationship to Abraham. But the blood of Jesus Christ is the only blood that can save!

Jesus told about the foolish young women who were counting on going to a wedding. But they weren't prepared. They had no oil in their lamps. They had not given their lives over completely to the control of the Holy Spirit.

I wonder if Jesus, as He told these stories, was not thinking of the day when He will prepare a great welcoming feast for His children. And that feast, that banquet in the City of God, will be no parable. It will be very, very real!

I like to try to picture it. A great table of pure silver, many miles in length. Weighted down with delicacies beyond our imagination. Fruit. Nuts. Almonds, figs, pomegranates, grapes. And fruits that we have never tasted. The fruit of the tree of life. Fruit so invigorating, so delightful, so much to be desired—because endless life is in it. But imagination fails!

I'm very sure, however, that some things will *not* be on that table. Ash trays and intoxicating drinks, for instance, would seem grossly out of place. Would Jesus provide for His people, with their new bodies, that which blackened the lungs of their bodies here and sent many to their death? Would He provide drinks that would distort their impressions of that happy day? Would He set before His people that which has sent so many thousands out to hurt and wound and kill, without knowing what they were doing?

And tell me. In that land where the lion and the lamb will lie down together in peace, in that land where there will be no violence and no death, would there be on that spotless silver table the flesh of dead animals? Will there be any slaughterhouses in heaven? You decide!

Come with me back—I don't know how far back.

But picture, if you will, a council of Satan and his fallen angels. Their purpose? To discover the most effective way to ruin and destroy the human race. One plan after another is discussed and rejected as not destructive enough. And then Satan himself comes up with the winning idea. He will concoct pleasing beverages that dull the minds of men and cause them to lose control. He will aim at the mind. Because that means the will. And that means control. And control is what Satan is after!

You say it never happened? I believe it did!

It was a failure on the point of appetite, in the Garden of Eden, that brought sin and suffering and death to this planet. It was on the point of appetite that Satan tried to defeat Jesus. But thank God, Jesus won a victory that day that can be yours and mine!

It is on the point of appetite that Satan is bringing much of the world today under his control. And you and I are not as safe as we may think. For Satan has more than intoxicating drinks in his bag of tricks. He uses smoke. He uses chemical combinations. He even uses respectable things like sugar. Anything that will dull the mind and make the conscience and the will inoperative. Because a dull mind and an inoperative conscience cannot make clear and right decisions. And a man's decisions decide his destiny!

Do I mean that a man's appetite can keep him out of heaven?

Yes. The sad truth is that millions of men and women today would be desperately unhappy at that silver table loaded with the delicacies of heaven. They would not feel at home without the indulgences to which they are accustomed. And so they will not be there. Not because they were not invited, not because they were arbitrarily excluded, not because of any discrimination, but because they would not be happy there. By their own choices they have unfitted themselves for the atmosphere of that better land. They would rather be somewhere else—anywhere else. Heaven, to them, would be torture!

You see, the majority of men and women today would probably rate heaven as they would a vacation spot. They would ask, "Does it have everything I want?" And some would choose the beauty of the mountains, the wonders of God's new creation.

But others would look for bars and casinos and pinball machines and racetracks and X-rated movies and the hottest night spots. And heaven wouldn't even be in the running. They would far prefer Las Vegas!

And Jesus, although He gave His own lifeblood to make eternal life possible for every child of Adam, will not force that life on any man against his will!

Those seated at that gleaming table will have asked of heaven only one thing—"Is Jesus there?" Jesus is there. And that makes everything all right. The vigor of eternal life, the untainted air, the indescribable beauties of heaven, the silver and gold and precious stones in abundance, the songs of the angels, the companionship of the best from all the ages, the opportunities for unlimited travel to other worlds, a city home, a country home built by their own hands—all these are added attractions of that better land. They have chosen Jesus—and everything else has been added!

In those radiant faces are no marks of dissipation or fatigue. In their hearts is no hidden hurt, no nagging guilt. In their eyes are no tears. Their minds are filled with eager anticipation of the life to come—a life that will know no parting, a life that will never end!

Friend, do you want to be there? Do you love Jesus enough to make any necessary adjustment in order to be with Him? It will be worth it—worth it a billion times over!

One day a great chasm will be fixed between life and death, between happiness and despair. And no man will be able to cross it. But you can decide today, just now, which side of that impassable gulf you will be on!

Hope Gets You Through the Night

A witch doctor sticks pins in a wax image. Or he points a ritual bone at his chosen victim. And now the man is doomed. Friends and relatives forsake him. There is nothing to do but wait for the voodoo death that he is sure will come.

And come it does. Why? Does the witch doctor's mysterious hex actually have the power to kill? There is plenty of evidence that it can and does result in death. But is there some evil force, inherent or acquired, in the bone that is pointed at the victim? Not necessarily.

Then what kills the man who is cursed? Simply this. His life is snuffed out by utter, overwhelming hopelessness. He is convinced that he has been trapped, that there is no escape, that he will die. And he does die.

It is sometimes that way with animals who are trapped but otherwise unharmed. And it is sometimes that way with a patient whose doctor has diagnosed a fatal disease. The patient feels trapped—and just gives up. An autopsy may show a malignancy, but no reason whatever for the patient to die so soon.

In the world of witchcraft, of course, a hex can be reversed if a more influential shaman can be persuaded to lift the spell. And in the medical world, the patient may ask for a second opinion. The second physician, or surgeon, may tell the patient that new techniques and more sophisticated equipment might diminish the disease or even cure it.

"This," says one psychologist, "is a very powerful influence. It's called hope."

Hope is what you have to have to get through the night. Without it, it's hard to get your breath!

Now illness, the doctor's diagnosis, even the word that death may soon be turning into your driveway—these are not the only culprits that snuff out your hope and take your breath away. It may be a persistent, nagging guilt, the loss of a loved one, or some other hurt.

But whatever it is that is crushing out your hope, I would like to offer you a second opinion!

In the sixth century before Christ, so an ancient fable says, the Greek lyric poet Ibycus, on his way to the festival of music at Corinth, was attacked and killed by two robbers. But just as he was dying, he saw a flock of cranes flying overhead and called upon them to avenge his death. And the robbers heard him.

All Greece was shocked by the violent death of Ibycus, and the people urged the authorities to bring the offenders to punishment. But this seemed impossible, for there had been no witnesses to the crime.

A few days later, in Corinth, in a theater open to the sky, a huge audience sat spellbound. It so happened that the choristers were impersonating the Furies, as they were called—the goddesses of vengeance. And such a performance, considering the angry mood of the people, seemed uncannily appropriate. No one was aware that in that theater, on the top benches, sat the two murderers.

In solemn step the singers slowly advanced. They were clad in black robes and carried torches that blazed with flame. Their cheeks were pale as death, and in place of hair they wore crowns of writhing serpents. Their weird song of vengeance rose higher and higher until it paralyzed the hearts and chilled the blood of the hearers.

At that very moment a flock of cranes swept across the sky and passed low over the theater. Instantly, from those top benches, there was a cry of terror. "Look, comrade! Look! The cranes of Ibycus!"

Every eye turned in the direction of that telltale cry of guilt. The murderers had informed against themselves. The atmosphere of vengeance, and the sudden appearance of those ill-omened cranes—to them the harbingers of swift revenge—had been too much for them. They felt trapped. They just gave up.

And so the cranes of Ibycus have become synonymous with the truth that guilt will out.

Who of us does not identify in some way with this fable? Who of us, at some time, surprised by our own personal cranes of Ibycus, has not cried out in the darkened theater of the mind, "I am guilty"?

Guilt is the most persistent enemy of our inner peace. It refuses to be bypassed or ignored or talked away. It cannot be quieted, because the cranes of Ibycus keep flying over our heads.

Guilt, like loneliness, can suffocate the will to live. Some of you at this moment may feel so guilty, so doomed, so desperate, so alone that you cannot breathe.

And then—*hope gets you through the night*!

Hope gets you through the night because your guilt can be healed. It cannot be *wished* away or *reasoned* away. But it can be *washed* away in the blood of Jesus.

Your guilt can be forgiven. And forgiveness is the only ladder out of guilt. Said the apostle John, "If we confess our sins, he is faithful and just to forgive us our sins, and to cleanse us from all unrighteousness." 1 John 1:9, KJV.

Forgiveness is the costliest thing in the universe, for it cost the lifeblood of the Son of God to make it possible. Yet forgiveness cannot be purchased. It cannot be earned. It is a gift—not for the deserving, but for the undeserving. The words of the prophet are full of hope: "Though your sins be as scarlet, they shall be as white as snow; though they be red like crimson, they shall be as wool." Isaiah 1:18, KJV.

God forgave David, whose hands were stained with blood. He forgave Mary, who had fallen seven times. He forgave Peter, who had openly denied Him. He wants to forgive you—even you. Even me.

Hope gets you through the night because you are not alone. It is your Creator who says, "Fear not, for I have redeemed you; I have called you by name; you are mine. When you pass through the waters, I will be with you; and when you pass through the rivers, they will not sweep over you. When you walk through the fire, you will not be burned; the flames will not set you ablaze." Isaiah 43:1, 2.

And remember the words of Jesus? "Surely I will be with you always, to the very end of the age." Matthew 28:20.

Hope gets you through the night because angels are with you. Listen to this: "The angel of the Lord encamps around those who fear him, and he delivers them." Psalm 34:7.

Hope gets you through the night because joy comes in the morning. The night is long. The darkest part of the night is just before the dawn. But nothing can hold back the morning. It was David who said, "Weeping may remain for a night, but rejoicing comes in the morning." Psalm 30:5.

Hope gets you through the night because you can

live again–and your loved ones too. Jesus says, "I am the resurrection, and the life." John 11:25, KJV.

Jesus met death head on and left behind Him an empty tomb. And He says, "Because I live, you also will live." John 14:19.

That's why David could write his beautiful psalm that says, "Even though I walk through the valley of the shadow of death, I will fear no evil, for you are with me." Psalm 23:4.

Death is an enemy. But the moment of dying does not have to be a horrible moment of panic. It can be like a baby going to sleep in its mother's arms. And when you wake up, the first face you will see will be the lovely face of Jesus. The pain will be gone. The tears will be gone. The sting of death will be gone!

Hope gets you through the night because there is a better land beyond this day. God says through the prophet Isaiah, "Behold, I will create new heavens and a new earth." Isaiah 65:17.

The apostle John, in the last two chapters of the Bible, describes that wonderful land, the land that no pen and no imagination could ever adequately picture. He says that God Himself will dwell with His people. And listen! "He will wipe every tear from their eyes. There will be no more death or mourning or crying or pain, for the old order of things has passed away." Revelation 21:4.

Think of it! The old order of things gone. Tears and trouble gone. Heartache gone. The long night will be over. And the morning will be forever new!

And never again will anyone say, "I am tired." Or "I am sick." Or "I am afraid!"

Listen again to John's description: "Then the angel showed me the river of the water of life, as clear as crystal, flowing from the throne of God and of the

Lamb down the middle of the great street of the city. On each side of the river stood the tree of life, bearing twelve crops of fruit, yielding its fruit every month. And the leaves of the tree are for the healing of the nations." Revelation 22:1, 2.

The tree of life will be there, and no longer will we be barred from eating its fruit. And the water of life is there. On the very last page of the Bible is this invitation: "The Spirit and the bride say, 'Come!' And let him who hears say, 'Come!' Whoever is thirsty, let him come; and whoever wishes, let him take the free gift of the water of life." Revelation 22:17.

I want to echo that invitation. That better land can be yours—if you want it. And you can drink of that water of life. It's for anyone who is thirsty.

And the good news is this! You don't have to wait for that living water. You can drink now. Jesus offered it to the woman who came to Jacob's well with her waterpot one hot noon. Remember? And in offering it to her, He was offering it to you.

And so I say to you, whoever you are, Leave your disappointing wells that never satisfy. Stop trying to dig your own wells. Digging is thirsty work. Come and meet Jesus. Come and drink. And you need never thirst again!

San Francisco and the East Bay were in the grip of a heat wave. And it was camp-meeting time. In those days everyone lived and cooked and slept in tents at camp meeting. And tents were stifling in the heat. Even so, the campers had crowded into the big pavilion to hear one of their favorite speakers—Pastor Luther Warren. Among them was a mother with two small children. And of course they were restless.

Finally the charming little two-year-old fell asleep in her mother's arms. The older child was blue-eyed, with slightly curling blonde hair. The mother was eager to hear the message and tried patiently to help the child at her side to sit quietly. But it was so hot, and the folding chair was so hard. Soon came the inevitable request—a drink of water.

The mother waited, reluctant to disturb the sleeping child. Then suddenly the little girl pointed vaguely in some direction, "There's a man over there who has a drink of water!"

In those days it was not dangerous for a child to ask a stranger for a drink—especially at camp meeting. The mother gave her permission, telling the little girl to come back right away. Then she settled back and relaxed. Maybe now she could listen to the message.

Suddenly, with unbelieving eyes, she saw her small daughter walk right up on the platform and ask the speaker for a drink! She sat transfixed as she saw Pastor Warren stop and pour a glass of cold water from the pitcher that had been placed on the desk. And the child expressed her thanks by lifting her blue eyes to gaze into his.

If you ever knew Luther Warren, you would know that he didn't mind the interruption a bit. Instead, it gave him the perfect opportunity to talk about cool, invigorating, living water—on a hot, thirsty day.

Look, friend! There's a Man over there on that cross who has a drink of water! Living water! And you can walk right up to Him and ask Him for a drink. He won't mind being interrupted!

Jesus was dying that Friday afternoon. The guilt of the world's sin was crushing out His life. In all history there had never been a more important moment. And the thief on the cross beside Him interrupted His dying with a request.

What happened? The whole plan of salvation stopped and waited while Jesus answered the prayer of the repentant thief!

He will stop to answer *you*—at any time! You can walk right up and ask Him for a drink—and never thirst again! You can ask Him now!

And a new and living hope will get you through the night. Any night. Every night. From now to forever!